Weight Loss Motivation:

84 Proven Life Hacks To Lose Weight

Table of Content

Introduction

Modern life is stressful and time consuming. Many of us find that our health and fitness (which should logically be right at the very top of our priorities) is somehow shunted down to the bottom of the list. We end up using food as a reward or a crutch to get us through bad times, to provide the only moments of pleasure in an otherwise unsatisfying day or to deal with boredom and dissatisfaction. Meanwhile, our physical fitness declines to the point where exercise is an uncomfortable chore rather than something we enjoy, meaning we are even less likely to go out and get our bodies moving.

You have taken an important step towards changing this unhelpful mindset — you are sincerely motivated to become healthier and happier. Right now, you are full of good intentions to overhaul your diet and increase your activity levels, and you look forward to feeling better both inside and out. This book contains helpful hints, tricks and suggestions to keep you on course when you feel your motivation is flagging or your bad habits start to reassert themselves.

You may feel that you have tried and 'failed' in the past — this is not the case! Those previous efforts taught you what works for you and what doesn't and, armed with that knowledge, you are in the best possible position to make a success of your current endeavor. Many, many people have achieved their health and fitness goals, and you are about to become one of them.

Chapter 1 – Exercise

1. Don't assume that an expensive gym membership will 'force' you to work out regularly. In reality, it is more likely to waste your money. Before joining a gym for the first time, set yourself a routine of exercises such as situps, pressups and stretches that you can do at home (there are many free exercise videos available online) every other day and stick to it for three weeks. If at the end of this time you have managed to complete your exercise routines regularly, then go ahead and join a gym. If you have not, then perhaps the gym is not for you and you should look for another form of exercise.

2. Know yourself. Is committing to a regular exercise class going to make it easier to find the time each week, or are you more likely to find an excuse not to go at that particular time? Do you need to have a regular time set aside for exercise, or do you need something that can be slotted in to your life around other things? If missing a class means that you 'miss' the opportunity for exercise for that week, then you need to have backup strategies to keep you moving. Some people find that a fitness class makes them feel self-conscious or find the exhortations of the teacher annoying, whereas others really enjoy the motivation and sense of community. Work out what it is that suits you best — there is no right or wrong.

3. Find a way to make a walk part of your everyday routine. If you live within five miles of your workplace, walk there. This should take you around an hour and a quarter at a brisk pace — this is not an excessively long commute and you will find that you feel sharper and more alert when you start work.

4. There is evidence to suggest that exercise in the morning is the most effective at burning calories. It also means you are less likely to ditch your workout because you can't face it after a long day. If you can, exercise before breakfast, as this will force your body to mobilize energy from fat stores rather than food.

5. Try not to become obsessed with your scales. The results are too easily influenced by other factors such as dehydration and whether you've been to the lavatory recently. If you must, weigh yourself once a week for your 'official' weight and use any in between 'unofficial' weigh ins as motivation.

6. Take measurements of your bicep, thigh, hips and belly at the start of your plan. This is a more reliable indicator of changes to your body shape.

7. Weight training is essential. Lean muscle burns calories even when it is not being used, so the more you have the better (within reason). Don't worry about 'bulking up' — frequent repetitions with small weights will build tone, not bulk.

8. For weight loss, intensity of training is more important than time. Although gentle, regular exercise is important, try to also undertake three high intensity sessions three times a week — as little as ten minutes of exercise that leaves you exhausted can make all the difference.

9. You should aim to increase your fitness targets by ten percent each week. If this week you can run for ten minutes, then next week try to run for eleven.

10. If you have the money, consider having a short course with a personal trainer, He or she can teach you how to exercise effectively, be mindful of your body and it is very motivating to have another person involved in your fitness journey. Consider it as an investment in your personal wellbeing.

11. Small changes won't be enough by themselves, but they are a brilliant way to burn off a few extra calories — really do try taking the stairs instead of the lift, opt for a standing desk rather than sitting down and walk short distances instead of taking your car or public transport.

12. Some things that you wouldn't imagine as exercise can be brilliant calorie burners — for example, going out to a club and dancing for a few hours is just as good as a session in the gym. Clearing out an attic or garage will help you build muscle and improve flexibility. Look for opportunities in your life to get moving, even without structured exercise sessions.

13. Consider taking a cold shower first thing in the morning, especially after exercise. Although it may seem daunting, the cold water will sooth aching muscles, stimulate the blood flow and improve circulation. It is also a sure-fire way to wake yourself up!

14. If you keep getting a 'stitch' (a sharp cramping pain in your ribs when you exercise) then keep moving, but press your fist into the area and take ten deep breathes. The pain should slacken off within thirty seconds and you can get on with your workout.

Chapter 2 – Food

15. Be honest about how much you eat and when. Keep a food diary for a week, and write down *everything* that you eat — sugar in your tea, that single M&M your colleague offered you, everything. You may be surprised at how much food is sneaking in without you being aware of it.

16. The 'Red, Orange, Green' rule means that, at every meal, you should have at least one food of each color on your plate. This encourages you to consume a good variety of vegetables.

17. Try intermittent fasting. Build up predetermined periods of time without food — start with twelve hours, then go to eighteen and finally twenty. You should not go for longer than twenty four hours without eating, and make sure that you do not let yourself become dehydrated. This is not starving yourself — you are training yourself to wait for your food and experience true hunger.

18. Don't binge after your fast. Although you should view all foods as available to you, don't 'shock' your digestive system with too much high fat or carbohydrates, as these may lead to cramping and diarrhea.

19. Cut calories by cutting carbohydrates from your diet. There is no need to completely eliminate all forms — after all, that would mean no fruit or vegetables for the rest of your life. Instead, focus on removing processed and refined carbs from your diet. These include flour, rice, pasta and anything which is high in sugar. Instead, eat protein-rich meals with a high fiber content.

20. Steer clear of over processed foods. Even if two dishes have the same calorie content, unrefined foods make your body 'work' harder to get those calories and you will feel fuller for longer.

21. Get used to leaving food. As children we are often told to finish everything on our plates, and this can teach us to override feelings of fullness, only considering a meal to be 'over' when the plate is clear. Instead, teach yourself to leave a small amount on the plate — remember, it is just as much of a waste to eat food you don't really want than it is to throw it away.

22. Don't worry about eating animal and vegetable fats. The only fat to keep an eye on is dairy — it is very easy to consume a large volume of cheese or cream without receiving the 'full' signal from your brain that would be triggered by the same amount of animal fats. Make sure you don't each more than a matchbox sized piece of cheese (around 40g) per day.

23. Some people suggest that a teaspoon full of coconut oil eaten as a snack will help suppress your appetite.

24. If you like spicy foods, adding chili to your dishes can help you lose weight. The intense flavor is more satisfying, some studies suggest it can boost your mood, and the heat can raise your metabolism, meaning you burn calories faster.

25. Increase the fiber in your diet (which will keep you feeling full for longer as well as improving digestive transit) by adding ground flaxseed to salads and soups. It is also rich in Omega-3

26. High fiber foods are a brilliant way to consume fewer calories but still feel full. However, be careful of suddenly introducing a lot of fiber into your diet, as it can cause bloating, flatulence and diarrhea. Build up your intake gradually.

27. Eat from a small plate. This will help you regulate your portion size.

28. Get plenty of sleep. Try to stick to a regular bed time and make your bedroom free from distractions such as screens or work.

29. Plan your meals in advance. If you leave it until you are hungry to decide what to eat, you will end up overeating or overshopping.

30. Do NOT snack while preparing your meals. It is easy to 'forget' these stolen calories and they will also cut down your enjoyment of your meal.

31. Try to avoid eating out or grabbing food on the go. The modern world is a food-rich environment, and as soon as you leave your house, you will be bombarded with inducements to eat. Next time you are out, look around at how many adverts and food displays you see, and remind yourself that you do not have to consume them.

32. If you get a craving for a specific food, remind yourself that most cravings will pass in five to twenty minutes. Note the time, drink a glass of water and wait until the time is up.

33. Brush your teeth. The sweet flavor in your mouth will trick your brain into thinking you have eaten something and make you feel less hungry.

34. If you find yourself snacking, choose foods which you have to work for — for example, pistachios take longer to eat as you have to shell them individually.

35. Accept that hunger is a natural feeling that you can survive, rather than something frightening or dangerous. It is good to feel actual hunger but

often a desire to eat is triggered by something else — boredom, habit or a need for comfort or distraction. When you feel hungry, ask yourself whether there is something else going on at that moment. Perhaps you have just seen an advert for food, or perhaps you have got into the habit of always having a mid-morning snack. You can safely ignore these types of hunger and find another thing to do rather than eating.

36. Set aside some time every week to plan your meals and do some batch cooking to make healthy eating easier in the week ahead. For example, you could cook a large batch of brown rice, then portion it up and freeze it, or make a lentil soup and do the same.

37. Many articles and books will tell you that eating breakfast is a vital part of losing weight. However, this is only true for individuals who go on to eat high calorie foods out of uncontrolled hunger later in the day. If you find that skipping breakfast means you are reaching for a croissant by ten thirty, then you should probably plan for a more nutritious breakfast earlier in the day. However, some people simply can't face food first thing in the morning. If you are one of these people, then don't force yourself to eat something you don't fancy. Bring a nutritious 'breakfast' to work with you and eat that when you are truly hungry for it.

38. Consider eating only once or twice a day. If you are on a calorie restricted diet but still having three meals and two snacks a day, then you may find that you never feel truly satisfied. You move from one small meal to another, taking the edge off your hunger but never vanquishing it. Eventually, your willpower breaks and you binge on an attempt to feel full, and when you return to your diet it is with an increased feeling of weariness at the inevitable deprivation. If this sounds familiar, then consider having a 'window' in your day when you can eat whatever you want. This is a variant of intermittent fasting models — you will eat all your calories in one go which means that you feel satisfied after eating.

39.If you make large amounts of food, then put your portion onto your (small) plate and immediately divide up what is left into tubs for the fridge or freezer. Sit out of sight of the food — go into another room if possible. If it is sat on the side or table, you will find yourself picking at it or going back for seconds.

40.Chew your food. This is an old tip but an effective one. It slows down the rate at which you eat, giving your brain more time to feel fuller.

41.Don't eat in front of the TV or at your desk. Concentrate on the food you are consuming and try to really enjoy it.

42.If you feel hungry, do something that will put you off eating. Clean the toilet, pull the hair out of the plug hole, empty the cat's litter tray or just visualize something you find unpleasant or disgusting.

43.Eat from a blue plate and put a blue cloth on your table. A study showed that people were likely to consume fewer calories when surrounded by the color blue rather than red or yellow.

44.Eat with chopsticks. People tend to eat more slowly and take smaller mouthfuls than when eating with a knife and fork.

45.When you treat yourself to high-calorie foods or snacks, take time to really savor them. Don't just wolf down a chocolate bar in a few seconds. Smell it, chew each piece, roll it round your mouth and concentrate on the sensations. You are likely to feel more satisfied than if you ate it more quickly.

46.Carry some healthy snacks with you, such as fruit or unsalted nuts. If you feel hungry you can dig into those rather than having to find something on the go, which may have a much higher calorie count.

47.Make sure that at least half your plate is taken up with fresh vegetables. You should also eat a palm-sized serving of protein — if there is any room left, you can add starches such as rice or potatoes.

48.Wait until your stomach rumbles before you eat. This will make sure that you are eating out of true hunger, not psychological needs.

49.If you feel hungry, sniff something pepperminty. This is thought to trick the brain into thinking you've eaten.

Chapter 3 – Drinks

50. Make sure you drink plenty of water. The amount of water you need varies from person to person and day to day depending on things such as activity levels and ambient temperature — there is no fixed 'eight glasses a day' amount that is right for everyone. The best way to check if you need to drink more water is by monitoring your urine. It should be a pale straw color with no or very little odor. If you find that your urine is darker, seems 'thick' or has a noticeable smell, you probably need to drink more water. If you are frequently passing large volumes of completely colorless urine, then you probably need to drink less.

51. At the start of the day, fill a two liter bottle with water and keep it with you to encourage you to drink. There is no need to spend money on expensive mineral waters — tap water is just as good for you. In fact, some mineral waters can be surprisingly high in sodium.

52. Be careful of 'sports drinks'. Although these can be of use to athletes on race day, they are often loaded with sugar and unnecessary electrolytes. Similarly, unless you are a professional athlete or have just run a marathon, you are unlikely to need to 'refuel' with the latest fashionable drink like coconut water or similar.

53. Steer clear of high-sugar drinks — this includes fruit juices and smoothies in which the fruit fiber has been removed. Not only do they contain unnecessary calories, but they will also cause a spike in your blood sugar that can lead to further hunger.

54. Opinion is sharply divided on the health risks of diet sodas and drinks containing zero-calorie sweeteners. It is best to try to eliminate or reduce the amount you consume.

55.Alcohol has empty calories. Try to avoid dark drinks (such as beer and red wine) or anything that has been sweetened (many liqueurs and bottled premixed 'alcopops' are very high in sugar) and stick to clear spirits with sugar-free mixers or dry white wine.

56.Many people swear by caffeine to help regular their food intake. While it is true that caffeine acts as an appetite suppressant, you should be careful not to drink too much, as it can give you headaches and lead to difficulties sleeping. Remember as well that adding milk and sugar will increase the calorie count dramatically — there can be as much as three hundred and eighty calories in a large latte with vanilla syrup.

57.Alcohol is also likely to lower your resistance to high-calorie foods, either on the night or the morning after. If you're going for a night out and know that you are at risk of a kebab on the way home or a fry-up to ease your hangover, plan in advance to have something more healthy waiting for you in the fridge when you get home to help you resist the urge.

58.Restaurant portions are notoriously large. Consider ordering two starters and ask for one to be brought instead of a main course, or offer to split a main with another member of your party. You can also ask for some of your food to be boxed up to take home with you. Just make sure that you mentally decide before you start eating which bits you will save — cut your pizza or steak in half straight away and do not touch the half you want to save.

59.Ready prepared 'low fat' or 'diet' foods are not always the healthiest choice. Read the labels to check the salt, sugar and additives contained in the product — manufacturers often put these in to boost the taste.

Chapter 4 – Gadgets and Gizmos

60. There are lots of apps on the market that will help you to track your exercise and calorie intake. One of the most popular is MyFitnessPal, which allows you to scan in the codes of food you purchase directly to your phone. However, there may be another one that you prefer — but make sure it is on a device that is convenient for you. Many people choose their smartphones, but this may not be best for you if, for instance, you work in an office where phones must be kept switched off.

61. Get a pedometer that will track your steps. Aim to complete ten thousand steps a day. The great thing about this is every little counts, so it's an encouragement to make journeys as short a few yards.

62. There are also many free podcasts that you can use to help with your training. Some of the most common are 'couch to 5km' ones, which guide you through intervals of running and walking, gradually building up until you can run continuously for half an hour. One of the best is getrunning, which allows you to play your own music rather than having to listen to the choice of the podcaster.

63. For many people, music is an essential motivator when exercising. There are many commercially available albums of music to exercise by, but you can also make your own playlists, using whatever motivates you. And you don't have to stick to music — some people find books on tape or talk radio a good way to entertain themselves on long runs.

64. BMI is a better way to measure your progress than straightforward weight, but even better is to be able to measure your percentages of

muscle and fat. Scales which will do this are commercially available, although can be pricey.

65. Getting a fitness buddy does not exactly count as a 'gadget', but is one of the best ways to stay motivated. You can team up for regular exercise sessions, join a weight loss group or have a shared goal such as a run or triathlon that you will undertake together.

66. The only exercise gear you really need is a good pair of running shoes, and (if appropriate) a decent sports bra. You can buy yourself other tops and leggings as you go along, but don't feel that you need a complete wardrobe of fashionable exercise wear before you can get out there.

67. Make sure you have comfortable shoes. This goes double for any shoes you exercise in, but consider your day to day footwear. If you regularly wear shoes that rub, pinch or have very high heels then you will feel less inclined to move around during the day, and will not feel much like exercising in the evening. Your footwear is supposed to protect your feet, not damage it — there is no need to keep uncomfortable shoes in your closet.

Chapter 5 – Supplements

68. A balanced diet should contain all the vitamins and minerals you need — it is actually very rare for a person who has access to a First World diet to have any deficiencies at all . However, if you are on a restricted diet, you may choose to top up with a broad spectrum multi vitamin to be on the safe side.

69. All herbal or homeopathic weight loss pills that you can buy over the counter are a waste of money. At best, they are laxatives, and most have no effect whatsoever.

70. Be careful with fat binders. Although these can be effective in supporting weight loss, they are well known for having very unpleasant side effects and can lead to vitamin loss as fat-soluble vitamins such as A, D, E and K are stripped out of your body.

71. Don't buy weight loss pills over the internet. You have no way of knowing what you will receive — people have died from taking unregulated medications.

72. Remember, a safe, effective weight loss pill is the holy grail of modern pharmaceuticals. When it's found, the world will know about it, and you will read about it on the front page of every newspaper. You will *not* stumble across it via some obscure website.

Chapter 6 – Motivation and Reward

73. Find ways to reward yourself without food — it could be a relaxing bath, some new clothes or time spent doing a hobby.

74. Have a specific, measurable goal that you want to achieve. This could be fitting back into your jeans, dropping a dress size or being able to run for five miles. Break this main goal down into smaller stages and write them down somewhere you can refer to them. Reward yourself when you reach each milestone.

75. Do something nice for your body. Get a massage, try dry brushing, or give yourself a pedicure. Rather than focusing on what you want to change about yourself all the time, remind yourself that your body is wonderful and amazing, and worthy of care.

76. Find your own weight loss mantra. This is something you repeat to yourself to help your motivation. Make it something positive rather than self-loathing or aggressive —what about 'It takes a million little victories' or 'I am feeling healthy, focused and determined'.

77. It takes around three thousand five hundred calories to build a pound of body fat. So if you have overeaten and feel that you have undone all your hard work, don't beat yourself up. It is very unlikely that one meal 'off diet' will completely sabotage your progress. More important is how you behave the next day — this is when you can get back on your diet and carry on.

78. Most people only consider how they feel before and during eating junk food, not how they feel an hour afterwards. This is why you keep coming

back for it — all your body remembers is the pleasure at the time, not the thirst, nausea or sluggishness afterwards. Next time you have too much sugar or end up with a Macdonald's, concentrate on how you feel an hour after eating it. Try to link those bad feelings in your mind with the food itself — next time, you'll be much less tempted.

79. Some people recommend having a 'fat' picture of yourself somewhere prominent — the fridge is a popular choice. However, it is even more motivating to have a picture of yourself looking your best as something to aim for, rather than one that makes you feel shamed and worthless. Pick a great picture of you or someone you admire looking fit and slim, and aim for that.

80. Keep your language about your journey to health positive. Avoid using phrases like 'I'm not allowed to eat xyz' or 'I hate being so fat'. Instead, use the language of success and empowerment by saying things like 'I'm choosing not to eat xyz at the moment' and 'I'm really looking forward to feeling more healthy'.

81. Think of ways to make social occasions more active. Often we end up seeing our friends in a sedentary setting, such as a bar or restaurant. Instead, make one social event per week into an active one — go for a walk, meet in the park or visit a museum or shopping center together.

82. Always order the smallest version of everything when eating out. Get a kids-sized meal, ask for a six inch sub and never, ever 'go large'. Studies show that we eat what is put in front of us and are likely to feel just as satisfied with the smaller portion as the larger one.

83. Don't feel bad about refusing food. There are likely to be many situations in which you eat to be polite or to celebrate rather than out of true hunger. A good example is in offices where it is the convention to bring in cakes or biscuits on a Friday afternoon, or on someone's birthday. Practice some

polite but firm phrases such as 'That looks lovely, but none for me, thanks' or 'Actually, I really fancy a cup of tea. Can I get anyone else one?' and then remove yourself from the situation.

84. Watch out for 'saboteurs'. If anyone pushes you to eat more than you want to, get them on board with your fitness and weight loss journey and be polite but firm. Remember, you are not depriving anyone else of a good time by becoming more healthy yourself, nor are you somehow criticizing their lifestyle choices. This is about YOU.

Conclusion

We hope that you enjoyed this guide to improving your health and fitness. You have taken an important step on a journey towards a happier, stronger you and you are now armed with the knowledge to make it to your destination. Remember to celebrate along the way, and take a moment to think about how far you've come and the progress you've made. Health and fitness is one of the most important gifts in the world, and only you have the power to give it to yourself. You deserve to be the happiest, healthiest you that you can be — go out there and get it!